I0789613

Table of Contents

DIET AND DIABETES: A PLANT-BASED DIET FOR THE PREVENTION AND TREATMENT OF TYPE 2 DIABETES

Diabetes is a condition that impairs the body's ability to process blood glucose, otherwise known as blood sugar.

Three major diabetes types can develop: Type 1, type 2, and gestational diabetes.

Type I diabetes: Also known as juvenile diabetes, this type occurs when the body fails to produce insulin. People with type I diabetes are insulin-dependent, which means they must take artificial insulin daily to stay alive.

Type 2 diabetes: Type 2 diabetes affects the way the body uses insulin. While the body still makes insulin, unlike in type I, the cells in the body do not respond to it as effectively as they once did. This is the most common type of diabetes, according to the National Institute of Diabetes and Digestive and Kidney Diseases, and it has strong links with obesity.

Gestational diabetes: This type occurs in women during pregnancy when the body can become less sensitive to insulin. Gestational diabetes does not occur in all women and usually resolves after giving birth.

Diabetes Basics

Type 2 diabetes often goes hand-in-hand with unhealthy cholesterol levels. Even someone with diabetes who has good control of their blood glucose is more likely than otherwise healthy people to develop any or all of several cholesterol problems that increase the risk of atherosclerosis and other cardiovascular problems.

If you have diabetes, you've already made changes to your diet and lifestyle that are targeted to keeping your blood glucose (blood sugar) levels steady. But given the increased risk of heart problems associated with diabetes, you may want to also take steps to keep your cholesterol levels steady as well.

Aspects of Cholesterol Problems

In and of itself, cholesterol is not a bad thing: It's present in every cell in the body and does a lot of good—supporting the production of hormones, digestion, and converting sunlight into vitamin D. Approximately 75 percent of the cholesterol present in the blood is produced by the liver, but the rest is derived from the diet, which is why making dietary changes is an effective way to keep cholesterol levels healthy.

There are two types of cholesterol:

- Low-density lipoprotein (LDL) cholesterol is regarded as "bad cholesterol." It's the soft, waxy stuff that can accumulate in the bloodstream and interfere with the flow of blood.

- High-density lipoprotein (HDL)—the so-called "good cholesterol"—helps keep blood vessels clear by carrying LDL cholesterol to the liver for disposal.

In addition to cholesterol, the levels of triglycerides (fats) in the body are important to heart health and so usually are considered a key aspect of a person's overall blood cholesterol "profile."

If you have diabetes, it can be hard to figure out how to eat to feel your best and keep your blood sugar under control. But there are lots of diabetic diet-friendly foods you can enjoy. And rather than keeping the focus on what foods to avoid with diabetes, it's refreshing to focus on the foods you can and should be eating more of. These top foods to eat with diabetes are nutrient-packed powerhouses that can help you control your blood sugar and stay healthy.

Research shows that plant-focused eating offers clearly positive outcomes for people with diabetes – with reductions in blood sugar, lipids and body weight. And for you naysayers who cringe at the thought of moving toward a plant-based eating plan, you may change your mind after reading this.

PLANNING A PLANT-BASED DIABETES DIET

A diabetic diet doesn't have to be complicated and you don't have to give up all your favorite foods. The first step to making smarter choices is to separate the myths from the facts about eating to prevent or control diabetes. If you're eating mostly or only fruits, vegetables, nuts, beans, whole grains, and meat substitutes like soy, you may cut your odds of getting heart disease, high cholesterol, high blood pressure, and type 2 diabetes, compared to a diet that includes a lot more meat.

There are many different types of plant-based diets. The three most common ones are:

Vegan : No animal products such as meat, eggs, or dairy products.

Lacto-vegetarian: No meat or eggs, but dairy products are OK.

Lacto-ovo-vegetarian: No meat, but dairy products and eggs are OK.

You can eat a plant-based diet without going completely vegetarian.

There are many ways eating more plant-based foods benefits people with diabetes:

- Better blood sugar management

- Improved heart health

- Weight loss

- Lower lipid levels

When we're speaking of plant-based, it's not all or nothing. I'm a believer in taking small steps to achieve the big goals of getting blood sugar readings in target range and improving overall good health. Moving toward a plant-based eating plan can start with simply adding more veggies to one meal per day or "going vegetarian" for one meal per week.

This Book provides dietary approaches and two healthful 7-day meal plans that are suitable for people on a calorie-controlled diet. One provides 1,200 calories per day and the other provides 1,600 per day.

Healthy Eating Guidelines

Managing both diabetes and cholesterol levels is a matter of being careful about the amounts of carbohydrates, cholesterol, and saturated fats in your diet, as well as making sure you're getting enough of certain nutrients that can help to improve your blood sugar and cholesterol levels.

Total Carbohydrates

There are several types of carbs: Of particular importance are complex carbs (a.k.a. starches), found in foods like legumes, whole grains, starchy vegetables, pasta, and bread, and simple carbs. Simple carbs are, simply, sugars.

For most people with diabetes, especially those who take insulin and are monitoring their blood sugar levels before and after meals, there's no hard-and-fast number of ideal carbs per day: That will depend on the results of each meter reading.

However, according to the National Institute of Diabetes and Digestive and Kidney Diseases (NIDDK), the recommended carbohydrate intake for most people is between 45 percent and 65 percent of total calories from carbohydrates, with the exception of those who are physically inactive or on low-calorie diets.

How to Make the Switch

Start eating more fruits, vegetables, beans, whole grains, nuts, and seeds. Depending on how far you want to take it, you can cut back on animal products, or cut them out.

Check with a dietitian to make sure you're getting the nutrients you need. For example, you'll need to take a supplement or look for foods fortified with vitamin B12 if you totally cut out animal products. You'll also want to check on whether you're getting enough iron, calcium, and zinc.

If you decide to swap dairy products for rice milk, nut milk, soy milk, or other plant-based alternatives, check the label to see how much calcium and vitamin D you're getting.

To get enough protein without meat, favor beans, lentils, nuts, seeds, □uinoa, or tofu.

You'll still need to stick with your doctor's guidelines about fat, calories, sugar, and salt. It's possible to get too much of those whether you eat animal products or not.

In the past few years, much of what we thought we knew about diabetes has been turned on its head. New understanding of the nutritional causes of diabetes gives us the power to keep it from occurring or to turn it around.

Here is what is supposed to happen: Our bodies turn starchy and sugary foods into glucose for our muscle cells to use for fuel. Insulin, a hormone made in the pancreas, ushers glucose into the cells.

People with type 2 diabetes, the most common type, generally have enough insulin. However, their cells become resistant to it, leaving too much glucose in the bloodstream, where it can cause problems.

Over the short run, people with uncontrolled diabetes may feel tired and thirsty, urinate fre□uently, and notice blurred vision. In the long run, they are at risk for heart disease, kidney problems, vision loss, nerve damage, and other difficulties.

DIETARY APPROACHES TO DIABETES

Diabetes diets typically call for portion control, carbohydrate limits, and for those who are overweight, calorie restrictions.

Fortunately, there is another way. Low-fat, plant-based diets are ideal for diabetes and the conditions associated with it, such as heart disease, weight gain, high cholesterol, and high blood pressure. And they offer the advantage of not requiring any weighing or measuring of portions.

The old approach recommended cutting down on carbohydrates. It's true that overly processed carbohydrates—those made with sugar or white flour, for example—are poor choices. However, delicious unprocessed or minimally processed foods, such as potatoes, rice, oats, beans, pasta, fruit, and vegetables, were the main part of the diet in countries where people were traditionally fit, trim and where diabetes was rare. Unfortunately, highly processed carbohydrates and affordable meat and cheese dishes have moved in, and now we have a worldwide type 2 diabetes epidemic.

A low-fat vegetarian approach recognizes that whole-food carbohydrates are fine; it's the fat in our diets that is the problem.

New information suggests that fat in animal products and oils interferes with insulin's ability to move glucose into the cells.

Eating less fat reduces body fat. Less body fat allows insulin to do its job. However, choosing skinless chicken, skim milk, and baked fish is not enough of a change for most people to beat diabetes.

The new approach eliminates fatty foods and animal protein, such as meats, dairy products, and oils, and offers unlimited grains, legumes, fruits, and vegetables. One study found that 21 of 23 patients on oral medications and 13 of 17 patients on insulin were able to get off of their medications after 26 days on a near-vegetarian diet and exercise program.

During two- and three-year follow-ups, most people with diabetes treated with this regimen have retained their gains.

The dietary changes are simple, but profound, and they work.

A study conducted by the Physicians Committee for Responsible Medicine with the George Washington University and the University of Toronto, looked at the health benefits of a low-fat, unrefined, vegan diet (excluding all animal products) in people with type 2 diabetes.

Give It a Three-Week Trial

1. Build Your Meals From the Power Plate.

It's not complicated! Fill your plate with whole grains, legumes (beans, lentils, peas), fruits, and vegetables. Drink water.

Keep nuts or seeds to a small handful once a day.

2. Begin a Vegan Diet: Avoid Animal Products.

A vegan diet has no animal products at all: no red meat, poultry, pork, fish, dairy products, and eggs. Why? Animal products contain saturated fat, which is linked to heart disease, insulin resistance, and certain forms of cancer. They also contain cholesterol and, of course, animal protein. It may surprise you to learn that diets high in animal protein can aggravate kidney problems and calcium losses. All the protein you need can be found in whole grains, legumes, and vegetables.

3. Avoid Added Vegetable Oils and Other High-Fat Foods.

Although vegetable oils are healthier than animal fats, oils are not health foods. All fats and oils are high in calories; 1 gram of any fat or oil has 9 calories, while 1 gram of carbohydrate has only 4 calories. The amount of fat we really need each day is □uite small and comes packed inside the Power Plate vegetables, grains, and beans.

Avoid oily sauces and salad dressings and foods fried in oil. Limit olives, avocados, nuts, and peanut butter. Read labels, and choose mostly foods with no more than 2–3 grams of fat per serving.

4. Favor Foods With a Low Glycemic Index.

The glycemic index (GI) identifies foods that raise blood sugar more than other foods. High GI foods can also raise triglyceride levels. Fortunately, beans, oats, sweet potatoes, and surprisingly, white and wheat pasta are among foods that are lower GI champions. So are breads such as pumpernickel, rye, multigrain, sourdough, and tortillas. Lower GI cereals are bran cereals, muesli, and rolled or steel-cut oats. Grains such as barley,

parboiled rice, couscous, corn, and □uinoa have a low GI.

High GI foods to limit are sugar and sugary products, white and wheat bread, corn flakes, and puffed rice cereals.

5. Go High-Fiber.

Aim for at least 40 grams of fiber each day. Choose beans, vegetables, fruits, and whole grains (e.g., whole-wheat pasta, barley, oats, □uinoa). Aim for at least 3 grams of fiber per serving on labels and 10 to 15 grams per meal. Start slowly. Expect a

change in bowel habits (usually for the better). Gassiness from beans can be minimized with small servings and thorough cooking and, if a problem will get better over time!

A note on vitamin B12: Those following a diet free of animal products (and all adults over the age of 50) should take a B12 supplement to protect blood and nerve cells.

MEAL SUGGESTIONS TO PREVENT AND REVERSE TYPE 2 DIABETES

1.   **SOFT TACOS**: a flour tortilla filled with beans, lettuce, tomato, and salsa

2.   **FAJITAS**: lightly sauteed sliced bell peppers, onion, and eggplant with fajita seasonings

3.   **CHILI**: homemade or vegetarian boxed or canned versions

4. VEGGIE LASAGNA: low-fat tofu to replace the ricotta cheese, layered with grilled veggies.

5. VEGETABLE STIR-FRY: vegetables seasoned with soy sauce or other low-fat stir-fry sauce and served over pasta, beans, or rice

SNACKS

1. Fruits: Carrot, celery, or other vegetables with low-fat hummus.

2. Baked tortilla chips with salsa or bean dip

3. Air-popped popcorn or rice cakes

4. Toast with jam

SOUP

Breakfast

1. **HOT CEREALS**: oatmeal with cinnamon, raisins, and/or applesauce

2. All-Bran or muesli with nonfat soy or rice milk and/or berries, peach, or banana

FRESH FRUIT

1. Pumpernickel or rye toast topped with jam (no butter or margarine)

2. Oven-roasted sweet potato home fries solo or smothered with sauteed mushrooms, peppers, and onions

2. Tofu scramble

LUNCH

1.   Mixed-vegetable salad with lemon juice, fat-free dressing, or soy or teriyaki sauce

2.   Legume-based salads: three-bean, chickpea, lentil, or black bean and corn

3.   Grain-based salads: noodle, couscous, bulgur, or rice

4.   Soups: carrot ginger, mixed vegetable, black bean, vegetarian chili, spinach lentil, minestrone, split pea, etc.

5.   Hummus spread on whole-wheat pita with grated carrots, sprouts, and cucumbers

6.   Black bean and sweet potato burrito with corn and tomatoes

7.   Sandwich made with fat-free meat alternatives such as barbecue seitan, Lightlife Smart Deli turkey style, or Yves veggie pepperoni slices and your favorite sandwich veggies

DINNER

1.   Pasta marinara: can be made with many commercial sauces

(any brand that has less than 2 grams fat per serving and is free of animal products)

2.   Beans and rice: black beans with salsa, vegetarian baked beans, or fat-free refried beans

3.   Pasta With Lentil Marinara Sauce (Meal Recipe)

MAKES 5 SERVINGS

1 pound pasta of choice

1 jar (26 ounces) fat-free, low-sodium, tomato-based pasta sauce

1 can (15 ounces) lentils, rinsed and drained

1/2 cup dry red wine (can be nonalcoholic) or low-sodium vegetarian broth, Salt to taste

Freshly ground black pepper

Cook the pasta according to package directions.

Meanwhile, combine the pasta sauce, lentils, and wine or broth in a medium saucepan. Heat gently and season with the salt and pepper. Serve over the drained pasta.

Per serving: 470 calories, 19 g protein, 91 g carbohydrate, 9 g sugar, 2 g total fat, 3% calories from fat, 0 mg cholesterol, 8 g fiber, 173 mg sodium.

4.   Cherry Tomato and Brown Rice

5.   Salad With Artichoke Hearts (Meal Recipe)

MAKES 6 SERVINGS

This delicious salad is a complete meal and is a great picnic or potluck dish. Because neither tomatoes nor rice benefit from refrigeration, it should be served at room temperature.

INGREDIENT

3 cups warm brown basmati rice

6 ounces marinated artichoke hearts, rinsed in hot water, drained, and sliced

1 cup chopped scallions

1 1/2 pounds red, yellow, or mixed cherry tomatoes, halved

1/2 cup chopped fresh basil

1/2 cup fat-free Italian dressing

3 tablespoons lemon juice

2 cloves garlic, crushed

1/4 teaspoon salt

Freshly ground black pepper to taste

1 head crisp lettuce

DIRECTION

- Place the rice in a large salad bowl and add the artichoke hearts, scallions, tomatoes, and basil. Mix gently.

- Combine the Italian dressing, lemon juice, garlic, salt, and pepper in a small bowl or jar. Whisk or shake until well blended. Pour over the salad and mix gently. Serve on beds of lettuce on individual plates.

Per serving: 153 calories, 4 g protein, 32 g carbohydrate, 3 g sugar, 1 g total fat, 6% calories from fat, 0 mg cholesterol, 4 g fiber, 376 mg sodium.

6.   Berry Mousse

MAKES 4 SERVINGS

This is so easy that it's hardly a recipe! Your blender does most of the work. This can be eaten as a pudding or used as a topping for fruit.

INGREDIENT

1 package (12.3 ounces) reduced-fat, extra-firm silken tofu, crumbled

2 3/4 cups thawed frozen unsweetened berries of choice

3 tablespoons sugar or 2 tablespoons agave nectar

1 tablespoon berry liqueur (optional)

DIRECTION

- Blend the tofu, berries, sugar or agave nectar, and liqueur, if using, in a blender or food processor until smooth.

- Spoon into 4 pudding dishes and refrigerate until chilled.

Per serving: 123 calories, 7 g protein, 24 g carbohydrate, 17 g sugar, 1 g total fat, 5% calories from fat, 0 mg cholesterol, 3 g fiber, 89 mg sodium.

7-DAY MEAL PLANS BASED ON 1,200 AND 1,600 CALORIES PER DAY

The ideal diabetes meal plan will offer menus for three meals a day, plus snacks. The two 7-day meal plans below, based on 1,200 and 1,600 calories per day, provide a maximum of 3 servings of healthful, high-fiber carbohydrate choices at each meal or snack.

NB: The meal plans are not based on complete Vegan Diet, each week has a calculated animal products which is not really a bad idea. You can also consider you doctor's guidelines on animal protein.

STEP BY STEP GUIDE

Measuring food portions can help with monitoring food intake more accurately.

A person with diabetes can enjoy a healthful, varied diet that helps manage their blood sugar levels. Developing this type of diet involves:

- Balancing carbohydrates, proteins, and fats to meet dietary goals
- Measuring portions accurately
- Planning ahead

1,200 CALORIE PLAN

MONDAY

Breakfast: One poached egg and half a small avocado spread on one slice of Ezekiel bread, one orange.

Total carbs: Approximately 39 grams

Lunch: Mexican bowl: two-thirds of a cup low-sodium canned pinto beans, 1 cup chopped spinach, a ⬜uarter cup chopped tomatoes, a quarter cup bell peppers, 1 ounce (oz) cheese, 1 tablespoon (tbsp) salsa as sauce.

Total carbs: Approximately 30 grams.

Snack: 20 1-gram baby carrots with 2 tbsp hummus.

Total carbs: Approximately 21 grams.

Dinner: 1 cup cooked lentil penne pasta, 1.5 cups veggie tomato sauce (cook garlic, mushrooms, greens, zucchini, and eggplant into it), 2 oz ground lean turkey.

Total carbs: Approximately 35 grams.

Total carbs for the day: 125 grams.

TUESDAY

Breakfast: 1 cup (100g) cooked oatmeal, three-□uarters of a cup blueberries, 1 oz almonds, 1 teaspoon (tsp) chia seeds.

Total carbs: Approximately 34 grams

Lunch: Salad: 2 cups fresh spinach, 2 oz grilled chicken breast, half a cup chickpeas, half a small avocado, a half cup sliced strawberries, one quarter cup shredded carrots, 2 tbsp dressing.

Total carbs: Approximately 52 grams.

Snack: One small peach diced into one-third cup 2% cottage cheese.

Total carbs: Approximately 16 grams.

Dinner: Mediterranean couscous: two-thirds cup whole wheat cooked couscous, half a cup sautéed eggplant, four sundried tomatoes, five jumbo olives chopped, half a diced cucumber, 1 tbsp balsamic vinegar, fresh basil.

Total carbs: Approximately 38 grams.

Total carbs for the day: Approximately 140 grams

WEDNESDAY

Breakfast: Two-egg veggie omelet (spinach, mushrooms, bell pepper, avocado) with a half cup black beans, three-□uarters cup blueberries.

Total carbs: Approximately 34 grams.

Lunch: Sandwich: two regular slices high-fiber whole grain bread, 1 tbsp plain, no-fat Greek yogurt and 1 tbsp mustard, 2 oz canned tuna in water mixed with a □uarter cup of shredded carrots, 1 tbsp dill relish, 1 cup sliced tomato, half

a medium apple.

Total carbs: Approximately 40 grams.

Snack: 1 cup unsweetened kefir.

Total carbs: Approximately 12 grams.

Dinner: Half a cup (50g) succotash, 1 tsp butter,

2 oz pork tenderloin, 1 cup cooked asparagus,

half a cup fresh pineapple.

Total carbs: Approximately 34 grams.

Total carbs for the day: Approximately 120 grams

THURSDAY

Breakfast: Sweet potato toast: two slices (100 g) toasted sweet potato, topped with 1 oz goat cheese, spinach, and 1 tsp sprinkled flaxseed. Total carbs: Approximately 44 grams.

Lunch: 2 oz roast chicken, 1 cup raw cauliflower, 1 tbsp low-fat French dressing, 1 cup fresh strawberries.

Total carbs: Approximately 23 grams.

Snack: 1 cup low-fat plain Greek yogurt mixed with half a small banana.

Total carbs: Approximately 15 grams.

Dinner: A two-thirds cup of Quinoa, 8 oz silken tofu, 1 cup cooked bok choy, 1 cup steamed broccoli, 2 tsp olive oil, one kiwi.

Total carbs: Approximately 44 grams.

Total carbs for the day: Approximately 126 grams

FRIDAY

Breakfast: A one-third cup of Grape-Nuts (or similar high-fiber cereal), half a cup blueberries, 1 cup unsweetened almond milk.

Total carbs: Approximately 41 grams.

Lunch: Salad: 2 cups spinach, a □uarter cup tomatoes, 1 oz cheddar cheese, one boiled chopped egg, 2 tbsp yogurt dressing, a quarter cup grapes, 1 tsp pumpkin seeds, 2 oz roasted chickpeas.

Total carbs: Approximately 47 grams.

Snack: 1 cup celery with 1 tbsp peanut butter.

Total carbs: Approximately 6 grams.

Dinner: 2 oz salmon filet, one medium baked potato, 1 tsp butter, 1.5 cups steamed asparagus.

Total carbs: Approximately 39 grams

Total carbs for the day: Approximately 133 grams

SATURDAY

Breakfast: 1 cup low-fat plain Greek yogurt sweetened with half a banana mashed, 1 cup strawberries, 1 tbsp chia seeds.

Total carbs: Approximately 32 grams

Lunch: Tacos: two corn tortillas, a one-third cup cooked black beans, 1 oz low-fat cheese, 2 tbsp avocado, 1 cup coleslaw, salsa as dressing.

Total carbs: Approximately 70 grams

Snack: One cherry tomato and 10 baby carrots with 2 tbsp hummus.

Total carbs: Approximately 14 grams

Dinner: Half medium baked potato with skin, 2 oz broiled beef, 1 tsp butter, 1.5 cups steamed broccoli with 1 tsp nutritional yeast sprinkled on top, three-□uarters cup whole strawberries.

Total carbs: Approximately 41 grams

Total carbs for the day: Approximately 157 grams

SUNDAY

Breakfast: Chocolate peanut oatmeal: 1 cup cooked oatmeal, 1 scoop chocolate vegan or whey protein powder, 1 tbsp peanut butter, 1 tbsp chia seeds.

Total carbs: Approximately 21 grams

Lunch: One small whole wheat pita pocket, half a cup cucumber, half a cup tomatoes, half a cup lentils, half a cup leafy greens, 2 tbsp salad dressing.

Total carbs: Approximately 30 grams

Snack: 1 oz almonds, one small grapefruit.

Total carbs: Approximately 26 grams

Dinner: 2 oz boiled shrimp, 1 cup green peas, 1 tsp butter, half a cup cooked beets, 1 cup sauteed Swiss chard, 1 tsp balsamic vinegar.

Total carbs: Approximately 39 grams

Total carbs for the day: Approximately 116 grams

1,600 CALORIE PLAN

Breakfast: One poached egg and half a small avocado spread on one slice of Ezekiel bread, one orange.

Total carbs: Approximately 39 grams

Lunch: Mexican bowl: a one-third cup brown rice, two-thirds cup home-made baked beans, 1 cup chopped spinach, a quarter cup chopped tomatoes, a □uarter cup bell peppers, 1.5 oz cheese, 1 tbsp salsa as sauce.

Total carbs: Approximately 43 grams

Snack: 20 10-gram baby carrots with 2 tbsp hummus.

Total carbs: Approximately 21 grams

Dinner: 1 cup cooked lentil penne pasta, 1.5 cups veggie tomato sauce (cook garlic, mushrooms, greens, zucchini, and eggplant into it), 2 oz ground lean turkey.

Total carbs: Approximately 35 grams

Snack: 1 cup cucumber, 2 tsp tahini.

Total carbs: Approximately 3 grams

Total carbs for the day: Approximately 141 grams

TUESDAY

Breakfast: 1 cup (100 g) cooked oatmeal, three-quarters cup blueberries, 1 oz almonds, 2 tsp chia seeds.

Total carbs: Approximately 39 grams

Lunch: Salad: 2 cups fresh spinach, 3 oz grilled chicken breast, half a cup chickpeas, half a small avocado, half a cup sliced strawberries, a quarter cup shredded carrots, 2 tbsp low-fat French dressing.

Total carbs: Approximately 49 grams

Snack: One small peach diced into one third of a cup 2% fat cottage cheese.

Total carbs: Approximately 16 grams

Dinner: Mediterranean couscous: two-thirds cup cooked whole wheat couscous, half a cup sauteed eggplant, four sundried tomatoes, five jumbo olives chopped, half a diced cucumber, 1 tbsp balsamic vinegar, fresh basil.

Total carbs: Approximately 38 grams

Snack: One apple with 2 tsp almond butter.

Total carbs: Approximately 16 grams

Total carbs for the day: 158 grams

WEDNESDAY

Breakfast: Omelet: two-egg veggie omelet (spinach, mushrooms, bell pepper, avocado) with half a cup black beans, 1 cup blueberries.

Total carbs: Approximately 43grams

Lunch: Sandwich: two regular slices high-fiber whole grain bread, 1 tbsp Greek plain, no-fat yogurt and 1 tbsp mustard, 3 oz canned tuna in water mixed with a quarter cup of shredded carrots, 1 tbsp dill relish, 1 cup sliced tomato, half a medium apple.

Total carbs: Approximately 43.

Snack: 1 cup unsweetened kefir.

Total carbs: Approximately 16grams

Dinner: half a cup (50 g) succotash, 1.5 oz cornbread, 1 tsp butter, 3 oz pork tenderloin, 1 cup cooked asparagus, half a cup fresh pineapple. Total carbs: Approximately 47grams

Snack: 20 peanuts, 1 cup carrots.

Total carbs: Approximately 15 grams

Total carbs for the day: 164 grams

THURSDAY

Breakfast: Sweet potato toast: two slices (100 g) toasted sweet potato, topped with 1 oz goat cheese, spinach, and 1 tsp sprinkled flaxseed.

Total carbs: Approximately 44 grams

Lunch: 3 oz roast chicken, 1.5 cups raw cauliflower, 1 tbsp salad dressing, 1 cup fresh strawberries.

Total carbs: Approximately 23 grams

Snack: 1 cup low-fat plain Greek yogurt mixed with half a small banana.

Total carbs: Approximately 15 grams

Dinner: Two-thirds cup quinoa, 8 oz silken tofu, 1 cup cooked bok choy, 1 cup steamed broccoli, 2 tsp olive oil, one kiwi.

Total carbs: Approximately 44 grams

Snack: 1 cup celery, 1.5 tsp peanut butter.

Total carbs: Approximately 6 grams

Total carbs for the day: Approximately 132 grams

FRIDAY

Breakfast: One-third of a cup Grape-Nuts (or similar high-fiber cereal), half a cup blueberries, 1 cup unsweetened almond milk.

Total carbs: Approximately 41 grams

Lunch: Salad: 2 cups spinach, a quarter cup tomatoes, 1 oz cheddar cheese, 1 boiled chopped egg, 2 tbsp yogurt dressing, a ⬜uarter cup grapes, 1 tsp pumpkin seeds, 2 oz roasted chickpeas.

Total carbs: Approximately 47 grams

Snack: 1 cup celery with 1 tbsp peanut butter.

Total carbs: Approximately 6 grams

Dinner: 3 oz salmon filet, one medium baked potato, 1 tsp butter, 1.5 cups steamed asparagus.

Total carbs: Approximately 39 grams

Snack: A half cup vegetable juice, 10 stuffed green olives.

Total carbs: Approximately 24 grams

Total carbs for the day: Approximately 157 grams

SATURDAY

Breakfast: 1 cup low-fat plain Greek yogurt sweetened with half a banana mashed, 1 cup strawberries, 1 tbsp chia seeds.

Total carbs: Approximately 32 grams.

Lunch: Tacos: two corn tortillas, one-third cup cooked black beans, 1 oz low-fat cheese, 4 tbsp avocado, 1 cup coleslaw, salsa as dressing.

Total carbs: Approximately 76 grams.

Snack: One cherry tomato and 10 baby carrots with 2 tbsp hummus.

Total carbs: Approximately 14 grams.

Dinner: Half a medium baked potato with skin, 2 oz broiled beef, 1 tsp butter, 1.5 cups steamed broccoli with 1 tsp nutritional yeast sprinkled on top, three-quarters cup whole strawberries.

Total carbs: Approximately 48 grams.

Snack: Half a small avocado drizzled with hot sauce.

Total carbs: Approximately 9 grams.

Total carbs for the day: Approximately 179 grams

SUNDAY

Breakfast: Chocolate peanut oatmeal: 1 cup cooked oatmeal, 1 scoop chocolate vegan or whey protein powder, 1.5 tbsp peanut butter, 1 tbsp chia seeds.

Total carbs: Approximately 21 grams.

Lunch: One small whole wheat pita pocket, half a cup cucumbers, half a cup tomatoes, half a cup cooked lentils, half a cup leafy greens, 3 tbsp salad dressing.

Total carbs: Approximately 30 grams.

Snack: 1 oz pumpkin seeds, one medium apple.

Total carbs: Approximately 26 grams.

Dinner: 3 oz boiled shrimp, 1 cup green peas, 1 tsp butter, half a cup cooked beets, 1 cup sauteed Swiss chard, 1 tsp balsamic vinegar.

Total carbs: Approximately 39 grams.

Snack: 16 pistachios, 1 cup jicama.

Total carbs: Approximately 15 grams.

Total carbs for the day: Approximately 131 grams

WEIGHT MANAGEMENT

There appears to be a link between diabetes and obesity. Many people with diabetes may be aiming to lose weight or prevent weight gain.

One way to manage weight is by counting calories. The number of calories that a person needs each day will depend on factors such as:

- blood glucose targets

- activity levels

- height

- sex

- specific plans to lose, gain, or maintain weight

- the use of insulin and other medications preferences

- budget

Various dietary approaches can help a person achieve and maintain a healthful weight, and not all of them involve counting calories.

FINAL THOUGHT

Managing blood sugar levels is key to living well with diabetes and avoiding some of its complications. Maintaining a healthful diet can help.

Following a diabetes meal plan can help make sure that a person is getting their daily nutritional needs. It can also ensure variety and help a person lose weight, if necessary.

In addition, a diabetes meal plan can help an individual keep track of carbs and calories and make healthful eating more interesting by introducing some new ideas to the diet.

No one plan will suit everyone. Ultimately, each person should work out their own meal plan with help from a doctor or dietitian.